M000086193

THE RENEGADE AUDIOLOGY MINDSET SHIFT

SEVEN MINDSET SHIFTS THAT WILL
SKYROCKET YOUR AUDIOLOGY PRACTICE

JARED M. BRADER, MBA
www.GreatAuDMarketing.com

KEITH N. DARROW, PH.D.
www.DrKeithDarrow.com

The Renegade Audiology Mindset Shift
Seven Mindset Shifts That Will Skyrocket Your Audiology Practice

ISBN 978-0-9993701-1-7

Cover design and interior layout by Five J's Design
Cover image adapted from original vector graphic by Ryzhi (Bigstockphoto)

THE RENEGADE

AUDIOLOGY
MINDSET SHIFT

SEVEN MINDSET SHIFTS THAT WILL
SKYROCKET YOUR AUDIOLOGY PRACTICE

JARED M. BRADER, MBA

DEDICATION

To the commitment, compassion, and empathy of every hearing care provider. May your heart and love for the profession continue to inspire the next generation of professionals.

To my patients, team members, and friends who inspire me to work hard, serve others, and Empower Active-Aging™.
Thank you for your commitment.

To my team at Intermountain Audiology.
Thank you for holding down the clinics.

To Keith.
The Journey Begins.

TABLE OF CONTENTS

PREFACE
Private Practice Audiology Must Be Totally Restructured

"I truly believe in positive synergy, that your positive mindset gives you a more hopeful outlook, and belief that you can do something great means you will do something great."
—RUSSELL WILSON

POLITICALLY-CORRECT AND WIMPY hearing care professionals, stop reading now. This book is not for those who emphasize being liked, who make excuses, or who want to bury their heads in the sand. The approaches outlined in this book are for an explicit kind of hearing care professional: **the Renegade Audiologist.**

To be clear, the term Renegade Audiologist refers to all people in the hearing health care profession, including Audiologists, Board-Certified Hearing Instrument Specialists, treatment coordinators, audiology assistants, technicians, front office staff, and many others. The Renegade Audiologist is someone who wants to be esteemed, who wants to help as many people as possible in their community, and someone who desires to be successful beyond their wildest dreams. This individual chose to work as a hearing health care professional to provide a life-enhancing impact on their patients, family, community, employees, and the professional community. These professionals are the champions of this book.

If you are reading this book, it is most likely because you are on a search for a proven method to revitalize your private practice; or maybe you or someone else believes that you need a little assistance converting your practice from where it is now to where you *want* it to be. It could be because you have noticed more competition in your area or a shifting industry landscape. You may have heard about my success in transforming the practices of hearing care professionals around the country who want to break free from the chains of dependency that accompany owning a private practice.

This book is my tell-all. It is my way of trying to help other hearing care professionals in private practice know more about me and the mistakes I have made, and to help them achieve the joy—and the financial freedom—that can come from an audiology private practice. This book is designed to be the first step, the 'intro' to my vault of newsletters and strategies that are required to build—on your own terms—the private practice of your dreams and to catapult your practice to extreme (and lucrative) success.

I want you to understand that I am an average guy from southern Utah with an unhealthy addiction to diet soda. (Hey, we all have our vices!) I loathe attention, I am not remarkably captivating, and I basically just want to achieve. I do not have any outrageous strengths or special gifts, but I am well-organized, I pay attention, and I learn from my mistakes. I have no formal education in audiology, I am not a Board-Certified Hearing Instrument Specialist, nor am I anything that even remotely resembles a hearing care provider—except for my heart. I have an MBA in Strategic Management and Marketing, and even more important than any degree, I have a knack for observing obvious problems in processes that most people engrossed in the day-to-day grind otherwise do not see.

In my 20s I took my grandmother to get 'hearing aid widgets.' Given my age and demographic, I really did not know much about hearing loss or hearing aids and what goes into it. Yes, like most red-blooded, breathing Americans, there were two things I knew: hearing aids are expensive, and they don't really work. (I look back now and realize that these common misconceptions could not be further from the truth.) My former college roommate and dear friend, Eric, worked for his father at the hearing center in downtown St. George, Utah, so, of course, I took my grandmother to my trusted friend to get hearing aids. While I was there, I was dumbfounded and awestruck; I wanted to fix everything wrong with the process.

Fast-forward several years and I now own that private practice and have catapulted revenue from a seemingly acceptable $437,005 per year to a growing audiology empire that brought in more than $8,706,885 in annual revenue in 2017.

I have learned many important lessons on my journey to building one of the fastest-growing, multi-clinic audiology practices in North America. Our post-recession growth has been 1,992%. I work no more than one day per week in my clinic. I spend the rest of my time being the family man I never thought I would be able to be, let alone have the resources to do well. I am able to take my girls to cheerleading and play practice, give my boys advice to help them get through the torturous high school years, and volunteer with the Sound of Life Foundation I created to give back to my local community in need of hearing health care.

It hasn't always been this way, however. In the last eight years, I have been poor and had the money run out (way) before the end of the month. In my early years as the man running the practice, I worked 90 to 100 hours per week, pulled an all-nighter at least once a week, and had the creditors knocking on the door. I've looked bankruptcy in the face, and I've had half my staff walk out on me over a disagreement. If that weren't enough, my brother, a Board-Certified Hearing Instrument Specialist, walked out on me and opened his own shop down the street from my practice!

Simply put, I am not happy with the status quo, and I won't accept complacency in my practice. I do not run my practice with an iron fist—in fact, completely the opposite; I manage my private practice with compassion, well-defined expectations, accessibility, accountability, and automation.

As a human, I am the furthest thing from perfect you will find on the planet earth. I have had the advantage and exceptional good fortune to have loving, supportive parents who were friend-like confidants and gave me a solid foundation to build upon. Before my 26th birthday, I had already owned three businesses and made every business mistake in the book. Over the last decade, as my friends were traveling, partying, and buying over-priced toys and adventures, I was building an empire, filing trademark applications, and fending off lawsuits of my own. I've enjoyed challenging the status quo and stirring the pot. I've been bitten in the ass a few times—I've had the state licensing board and consumer protection call my office after receiving complaints from other practices in my town. (Perhaps you would call them my "competitors," but I believe my only competitor is myself, not other practices, since I can only control what happens in my practice. More on this concept later in the book!) From the scars and battle wounds, sleepless nights, and stress, I've emerged victorious with systems and strategies that work. Period. (And I did all of this while providing an exceptional patient experience—yes, you *can* be a caring person with good intentions and still make money.)

These systems and strategies which we share with coaching clients all over this great United States of America are proven in our private practices and hundreds of others. Strategies that practice owners pay dearly for (some as much as $52,400 a year) to implement in their own practices. These systems can provide you with the future you have always dreamed of in private practice audiology—and in your private life. The same future you envisioned as a young student when you applied to school, or the first time you picked up an otoscope.

These systems we have developed work—but only if you commit to the mindset shift. Respectfully, the letters after your name, your certifications, and your accolades do not matter. Combining your passion, your drive, your commitment to your practice, and your commitment to using our systems will change your life. Forever. And most importantly, you will build a practice that can withstand any market disruptions that lie ahead (e.g., managed care, retail outlets, box stores, OTC, etc.).

If you acknowledge that the private practice audiology model needs to be completely restructured, this book is for you. If you believe that there is something drastically wrong with a clinical profession in which 80% of people afflicted with a disorder ignore sound medical advice to seek treatment, this book is for you. If you agree that 2–4% industry growth is actually a HUGE net loss when you consider how many people live longer healthier lives, this book is for you.

But if you think that what has enabled your practice to survive—not *thrive*—over the past five years will get you through the next five to ten years of big box stores, discount retail shops, managed care, and OTC hearing aids, then you are in for a shocking surprise, and perhaps this book *isn't* for you. Competition, third-party groups, volume retailers, and OTC hearing aids have been infiltrating the audiology market we enjoyed a few years ago. You may be shocked to learn that I actually welcome each of these players to the hearing health care field. Why? Because none of them can compete with me or my team, and they can't even come close to competing with our systems.

At a recent industry conference, a vendor had a Post-it wall for people to post their ideas about "what challenges lie ahead for the field of audiology." And all the usual suspects were listed: OTC, regulations, big box stores…blah blah blah. When I looked at the board, all I could see was hearing care providers whining, complaining, and burying their head in the sand to avoid the real problem: ALL OF US. Complaining won't help you one bit, and neither will the manufacturers. Getting serious about your future in this industry will. I believe it is better to seek out mentors, coaches, and have-done-its to provide you that guiding light on what to do and how to get it done. That is the aim of this book.

Don't envy those of us enjoying a liberated private practice lifestyle with complete personal and financial freedom. Join us instead. Join the Excellence in Audiology™ movement and enjoy the excitement and freedom that our member-clinics have come to find.

—*Jared M Brader, MBA*

INTRODUCTION
Establish Goals, Take Action, Continuously Progress

The path to success is to take massive, determined actions.
—TONY ROBBINS

I'M SORRY TO DISAPPOINT, but this book is not a marketing book. It is, however, the closest thing to a 'silver bullet' that will introduce you to a marketing system that works to bring unimaginable success to your private practice. Period.

This book was written for an explicit type of professional in the hearing care industry, one who spends myriad hours wearing many hats and recognizes that treating patients is most often the easiest part of the day. There are so many things that hearing care providers were never taught in school, things that have been wearing you down over the years, things that don't come naturally to most people that work in private practice audiology. I've spoken with countless Doctors of Audiology, university professors, Board-Certified H.I.S., people who teach the H.I.S. certification course, etc., and not a single one of them can explain, in any detail, how to succeed in private practice.

Following the approaches discussed in this book will help to radically change your outlook on private practice. In other words, if you commit to the mindset shift, if you consistently implement the systems discussed in the book, your practice will not only soar to new heights, but your personal freedom will have no restraints, and you will experience the freedom of running your own practice—not being run *down* by it. This innovative model will free you to serve others with passion, make much more money, and give generously to your employees and community, all while creating a remarkable legacy.

In this book I am going to challenge everything you have been taught—everything you have been programmed to accept as true—over your career and education. I urge you to take notes, highlight things that strike you, and write in the margins; but most of all, make sure to implement each concept into your practice with massive action. This is how you will change your personal and professional production. To help you in this, I have included blank notes pages at the end of each chapter so you can jot down your ideas and questions you would like to discuss in greater detail with my team of AuDExperts Certified Coaches.

In this book you will learn:

- **How to stop wasting your money** on marketing that doesn't work at a sustainable level—and never really has. You will learn to spend your money on wiser marketing methods, ones which will bring your business to newer and better heights.

- **How to keep your patients and referring physicians engaged** each and every month and change them into advocates who give you rave reviews.

- **How to be cautious of the industry consultant** who has not worked in a private practice in years—if ever.

Isn't it crazy how some people that 'advise' in this industry have never even seen a patient or had to pay a utility bill for a business they have owned? They will sometimes tell you that all your problems can be solved by doubling the number of new patients you take in. This simply is not so, not without implementing other strategies also. It simply doesn't work that way. If it did, I wouldn't need to write this book—and you probably wouldn't be reading it!

I have seen this play out in my own practice, and many other practices as well. Let me tell you, without the correct internal systems in place, you might as well flush your investments—marketing, time, energy, and money—right down the drain. I need you to commit now, before you read another page, to seeking out the ideal patients for your practice. If you want to follow advice that will help you double or even triple your numbers, you must commit to the system that will bring you the ideal patient and help your practice blossom. If, however, you think that everyone with a pulse and a hearing loss is your ideal patient, please stop now, and do not bother to invest in these systems. (Perhaps you can send the money you *would have* spent to my nonprofit Sound of Life Foundation so at least someone can benefit.)

A mentor, Dustin Burleson, once said to me, "Everyone is not a good patient for your business. You must determine a 'specific someone' for whom you are perfectly matched."

I want to teach you how I made my biggest mistakes in building my practice and how you can avoid doing the same. There are certain costly pitfalls you must avoid in order to make your practice soar. The steps you learn to take today will control how you address these issues in your practice, how much success you achieve, and how big you grow your bank account. I can guarantee that hearing care professionals who have retired with larger-than-life retirements, who live life on their own terms, have all dodged these mistakes in their own practices. You will learn how to avoid the foreseeable absurdity that runs rampant in our industry by electing to tackle this challenge head-on.

In addition, you will receive the perfect formula for creating compelling content that will attract the right patients to your practice. The bottom line is that your patients do not want to be jaded or lulled into action. The thing is, they actually want to be *wowed*! So many professionals disregard this piece of advice to their own peril. On my very first day of private coaching with new clients, I can tell within five minutes if they are approaching my tactical issues properly or not. Fixing certain problems is really very simple and can generate a multi-million-dollar swing in their practices. If I told you to fly to St. George, Utah, and make a million dollars or more over the lifetime of your practice within the first five minutes, you would probably tell me that it is impossible. The truth is, though, that it *is* possible. We do it every day for our clients who take that massive action of applying our systems on their road to an improved, greater, and brighter future.

There are five key mistakes to avoid in your practice marketing. If you can correct these, your return on investment will hit the roof, right past the tiny industry average. The average investment in marketing for a typical audiology practice in 2015 was $63,458. Unfortunately, even that minor investment was undoubtedly wasted. Blindly copying marketing and advertising strategies of big retailers or non-marketer competitors will not make you rich. Here's a tip: **never use a manufacturer's marketing piece** (unless you believe you're only as good as the widget you sell because every other practice in town has access to those very same ads).

And here is the good news. You don't need a $100 million budget to mess around with and try to fine-tune. Who wants to waste another penny on marketing this year, next year, or ever? Nobody does. **Well, the truth is, I have already done the testing.** This is my way of giving back and thanking you for allowing me to share my ideas and my proven results.

There is only one metric, or marketing KPI (Key Performance Indicator), you should worry about in today's economy and slow-to-no-growth profession of hearing health care and audiology. It is truly the big ticket to your imminent success. I promise you will cry tears of joy and relief when you finally learn how simple the concept is to implement. This joy will come from your newfound productivity and results.

I do warn you that you will likely be frustrated about all the wasted years when you *could have* been earning the rewards of these perfected strategies. But there is no looking back now; there is only moving forward with purpose!

With each strategy and concept outlined in this book, you have a chance to start anew. There are many average audiologists or hearing health care professionals that make excuses by saying things like, "That would *never* work for my practice." Some of the most intelligent doctors in the room ask, "How can this work for me?" Well, you can be the entrepreneur who turns over every stone, questions every tradition, and looks for ways these strategies can be effective in your practice. Start today, and get rid of the baggage that you have been carrying since you began. As I said, the profession of audiology that we hold so dear must be entirely re-designed. Yes, now is the time!

Come on, and let's get started!

ACTION ITEMS WHAT WILL YOU DO NEXT?

_____

_____

_____

_____

_____

_____

_____

_____

_____

_____

_____

_____

_____

_____

_____

_____

_____

_____

_____

_____

_____

_____

_____

_____

_____

_____

_____

_____

_____

_____

_____

_____

_____

CHAPTER ONE

Quit Believing It's All About You

"Those who are happiest are those who do the most for others."
—BOOKER T. WASHINGTON

THE FIRST SECRET TO SUCCESS in private practice is simple: **you can't do it alone.** As I said before, I've been where you are right now in your practice, wondering how you can do better. I too believed my education and my credentials were my tickets to success and that I was golden. Everything else would just be easy. Peaches and cream, right? Our success was guaranteed. No more worries, stresses, or failures. Keep reading because I'm going to explain why that way of thinking is totally incorrect. You've probably been humbled, as I have, by failures, by creditors, and by your patients.

It's really *not* about you.

The future is about much more than *you*, and if you only focus on yourself, you will never achieve the success you dream of. Never. As difficult as it may be, I urge you to accept this principle and get rid of the focus on you and/or your power as a doctor, health care provider, or practice owner.

Instead, you are going to learn to focus on the areas which really, truly matter. I guarantee that if you listen and apply, great things will happen. Commit to this, step aside, put your full attention on the areas of your practice outlined in this book, and you will yield insane outcomes.

I truly mean it when I say that it really isn't about *you*, but rather *everything* and *everyone else*. Let's begin with your staff. Developing a kick-ass staff that doesn't need to hang on your every word is the key to your freedom. You must be able to trust them fully with the responsibility of serving your patients with excellence. You must take constant steps towards building a business that will run smoothly without *you*.

Consider this question for a moment: how much attention do you place on your hiring process? Do you hire slow and fire fast?

Over the years as I have built my staff of 28, I've seen great people come and go. Honestly, the team that you surround yourself with can make or break your aptitude to achieve extreme success. If you think you can be all things to all people at all times, you are dead wrong. It doesn't work that way. During my consulting calls, as I evaluate, diagnose, and propose action plans with new clients (who pay a significant sum of money for this advice), I am capable of determining almost immediately whether I am working with a business where nothing at all is going to happen without the doctor's consent, vs. a business which is going to succeed and produce the kind of income you can only imagine.

The bottom line is that your practice needs to be able to run on autopilot. Today's audiology practices are complex. To assume that you can do everything is very naive. You simply cannot. And if you try, your results will be average and your stress high. You must have the correct individuals executing the correct jobs, without fail, and without direction. Each and every staff member must have the proper tools they need to do their jobs effectively. And if you want to generate a dependable system, they must be on the same page with your business goals and office procedures. You need to understand that it is your job to empower them with the responsibility to act and produce great results without your interference.

This is important. If you really want to change your revenue and success rate, you cannot do it on your own. Once you stop this way of thinking, you will see instant results in many areas of your private practice. The secret to leveraging your most expensive business expense (payroll) is building the right team and then treating them like gold. Do this, and you will see them rise to your expectations without fail.

One of the biggest mistakes I have seen in managing staff is a lack of expectations. Everybody in business tends to focus on the concept of 'accountability,' but without clear and achievable expectations, you can't hold anybody accountable (and each staff member can't be expected to hold themselves accountable).

During a recent on-site training, we asked each employee of the practice, "What is your daily, weekly, and monthly expectation of productivity at work?" We got some great answers—and some not so great answers—but not a single person (of the 20+ that were in the room) could actually quantify their expectations. As an example, the practice's best front office person said, "It's my job to keep the schedule full and the providers busy with patients." GREAT ANSWER! And despite the fact that she has been working at the practice for many years and is a valuable team member, even she couldn't answer the next question: "Well, how many new patients does your clinic need per week?" She had no idea how many patients. Keep in mind, this is a multi-clinic, multi-million-dollar practice.

Once you have learned how to inspire your staff, you will find that they are serving your patients with excellence, growing your practice, and getting results for you. You will also notice that they will constantly go above and beyond. Your projects will get completed quickly, your operations will run smoothly, and you'll be creating ecstatic patients who will spread the word about you and your amazing practice and how well you operate as a team, which will result in numerous word-of-mouth new patients. And the best part is if given the right motivation and the right tools to do their job, your staff can do it without *you* looking over their shoulder. This perfected approach is going to create a patient experience that encourages understanding, compassion, and absolute shock and awe in your practice environment. **Train your staff well, and then get out of their way.**

Hearing care providers are taught that patients come to us because they are seeking something very basic: restored hearing clarity. While that may be partially true, what they really want is somebody who understands their struggles, the impact hearing loss is having on their life and the lives of their loved ones, and their fears and worries about growing old. Our patients want to avoid the pain of isolation and aging. They want to be able to be a part of the conversation—and they don't want to be limited by background noise!

Many patients are fearful and apprehensive about taking that first step into your office for a hearing evaluation. Nowadays, even if you help your patient attain their goals (and more), if your employees do not make them comfortable and help them feel cared for and special, they will leave your practice indifferent and displeased. Regrettably, most of my new coaching clients are stuck in the mindset that they must make up for—or shoulder the load—for a weak staff. Most of the doctors I meet fail to invest their time to empower their staff and, hence, fail to bring an even greater patient experience. I'll say it again—you just cannot do it all! So, it's easy: stop trying, and focus on the *important* before the *urgent*. Not taking this crucial step immediately will actually hurt your results, not help.

Implementing this strategy immediately will have massive implications on your legacy as a professional and leader in your community. Your legacy, such as that of Steve Jobs,

WHAT IS YOUR TEAM'S M.O.?

Modus Operandi is the term used to describe how you get stuff done. Every person has their own M.O., and when enabled to harness their strengths, they put forth their full capabilities and produce amazing results.

WHAT IS CONATION?

The most significant word you have *never* heard is **conation**, which means "the aspect of mental processes or behavior directed toward action or change and including impulse, desire, volition, and striving." Conation is a mindful determination to carry out desired acts.

As Certified Kolbe Experts, my team can teach you to recognize the nature of inspired instincts and empower people to release the unlimited influence of their own natural predispositions—in other words, their Modus Operandi. This will enable you to:

- Improve Individual Production
- Improve Relationships
- Become Efficient Parents
- Launch Rewarding Careers

THERE ARE FOUR ACTION MODES YOU'LL WANT TO FOLLOW.

1 **FACT FINDER**—the innate way we gather/share information.
2 **FOLLOW THRU**—the innate way we arrange/design.
3 **QUICK START**—the innate way we deal with risk and uncertainty.
4 **IMPLEMENTER**—the innate way we handle space and tangibles.

TWELVE WAYS TO SOLVE PROBLEMS

The blend of the Four Action Modes defines 12 Methods of Problem Solving as can be seen in the image to the right. We can solve problems using any of the 12 methods, but each individual has four, one in each Action Mode, which permits us to do our most effective and inspired work.

It doesn't matter what four blends of talent we decide to use. Each individual will be extremely fruitful and receive a better sense of achievement when they work in their own unique mode. Remember that we make the biggest impact when we learn to solve problems in a way that is natural for us as individuals.

12 METHODS OF PROBLEM SOLVING

FACT FINDER	FOLLOW THRU	QUICK START	IMPLEMENTOR
SIMPLIFY	ADAPT	STABILIZE	ENVISION
EXPLAIN	MAINTAIN	MODIFY	RESTORE
STRATEGIZE	SYSTEMATIZE	INNOVATE	PROTECT

Walt Disney, Bill Gates, Warren Buffet, Richard Branson and Jeff Bezos is what you leave behind when you are gone. Each of the above entrepreneurs is either in the midst of creating or has already created a legacy that centered around empowering the individuals around them to become better than they ever thought they could be. Think about that for a minute. Are you, with your busy, packed days and crazy stressful life, implanting more confidence and making a greater impact in the lives of your staff then *they* could ever imagine? If not, remember that the best leaders do—and you should start today!

If you've never studied the success of Walt Disney, you should. He's a great example of one of the greatest business entrepreneurs of all time. His legacy of Disney demonstrates what imagination, inventiveness, and perseverance can do for a business empire. According to Forbes, Disney is one of the most recognized and valuable brands, and the company has over $55 billion in annual revenue with more than 195,000 workers. Walt Disney has left an amazing and lasting impact on the world with his legacy. And the money is quite impressive too!

Like Walt, Bill Gates, Warren Buffet, Richard Branson and Jeff Bezos are all in the process of leaving lasting legacies founded on their innovations and commitment to changing the status quo. Saying this is not to overwhelm you—your legacy doesn't have to produce billions every year in order to make a difference. That's not the point. You can, however, leave a legacy on the people you touch, and that includes your staff.

Consider for a moment the legacy *you* have always wanted to leave. Now go do these things and make it happen. It is so easy to get sidetracked while we are focusing our time, attention, and energy on other things that may seem urgent, but in reality have very little significance in the grand scheme of things. Begin now by emphasizing the important aspects which will shape your legacy for generations. Nitpicking *how* your team gets results and losing sleep because they don't do things exactly the same way you would, all the while utterly failing to measure the right performance indicators, is foolish.

Now is the time for you to change that—yes, right now! Therefore, the next step is quite simple. **Think about the legacy you want to leave, and take instantaneous massive-action steps to make it materialize.** Right now, you are probably thinking that this sounds a lot harder than I say it is. At one time, I wanted to control everything too. But trust me, the more you let go of control, the greater your results will be. Each time I slip up and begin to micromanage, I can see the results weaken (from both a revenue and morale standpoint). The more you let go, the better. Use your influence for good. Implement systems, teach your staff, delegate responsibility, set expectations, measure your performance correctly, and then celebrate or tweak the system. But do *not* interfere. That is one of the worst traits a hearing care professional can have as a practice owner.

In order to leave a legacy, you're going to have to focus on the big issues of our time, including:

- your core values

- how you build your team

- your place in the market

- how you are attracting patients

- what you say to prospective patients, and *how* you say it

- the degree to which your business structure is on autopilot, and how you make it more independent

The last item in the list is the central point you should focus on if you are to be successful in your practice and realize the level of success and freedom you desire.

Here is a recent example of this. One of my Renegade Audiologist friends asked me to fly to Boston for a golf fundraiser in the middle of the week. Many practice owners and audiologists in my position would not be able to do it because they are afraid their office would come to a standstill, their patients would go without care, or their office would simply fall apart in their absence. Not me! I hopped on a plane, flew across the country, and played a round of golf to benefit his hearing foundation. This was an enjoyable trip, and my offices were still open, changing lives, and paying for my trip.

Think about it. Could you do the same right now? Is your system built for freedom and autonomy in your absence? If not, it's time to make some serious changes.

Here's a story for you to mull over. I know personally how important this issue is because over the last eight years I have learned about it the hard way. I didn't always have the fabulous team I have today, or the office that runs on autopilot in my absence. In fact, I didn't even realize I had created such an autonomous system until the day a handful of my managers walked out on me.

It was December 2016 when my management team was satisfied with the status quo. They didn't want to take the next step with me to revolutionize our industry; they were content with what we had. The day your managers walk out on you is the day you will, without a doubt, learn that it is *not* all about you. It really isn't. The sooner you realize this concept and act to make it about your patients, your staff, and your family, the sooner you will be on your way to a higher level of success. When you make your staff a high priority, you will discover how it comes back to your practice and your patients. They will give their heart to help you reach your company goals.

I can't imagine having a practice where the providers think it's all about "being the doctor." The smartest audiology practice owners on the planet have realized they must lead a happy team, support their employees with opportunities for growth and responsibility with the practice, and then reap countless rewards from doing so. It doesn't work in reverse. If you are waiting for the day you have *massive* wealth to start treating your team like they are diamonds, you are doing it

DID YOU KNOW?

JetBlue and Southwest Airlines are the top two airline employers to have made it to the top 15 of Forbes 500 Best Employers?

Did you also know that Southwest and JetBlue Airlines are ranked number one and number two in customer satisfaction? And that these airlines put employer satisfaction ABOVE customer satisfaction (and rank shareholders lowest on their list of priorities)?

Coincidence? I think not. A representative of Southwest airlines said it best:

"We believe that if we treat our employees right, they will treat our customers right, and in turn that results in increased business and profits that make everyone happy."
—Southwest Airlines

Can you say the same for your practice?

all wrong. You will never achieve massive wealth that way; it's just the opposite. Your employees interact with patients every day, and they cannot and will not treat those patients like they are number one until you start treating your employees like they are number one.

I've interviewed hundreds of employees for our own practices and coaching clients, worked with dozens of hearing care providers, hired audiologists for my own practice and others around the country, and built extensive training programs for AuDExperts and Excellence in Audiology™ member-clinics to improve the human capital of our industry. This experience tells me that the single most important investment with the largest potential for leverage into unheard-of success is your investment in human capital.

Building a team of superstars that will care for your patients without being micromanaged is the ultimate goal. Train them on your system, encourage them, incentivize them, and get the hell out of their way. You should be the visionary leader and cheerleader of your staff, not the reason your practice is being held back.

In my coaching groups, the most successful hearing care professionals—those with the highest incomes, who have the most free time with their families, and who are in the early stages of building a legacy—all get this right; they make time in their schedules to *put people first.*

When was the last time you met with your team to help them visualize where your practice will be in three to five years? How often are you encouraging your employees to reach higher and grow deeper than even *they* thought possible? **The time to start is *now*.**

ACTION ITEMS WHAT WILL YOU DO NEXT?

_____

_____

_____

_____

_____

_____

_____

_____

_____

_____

_____

_____

_____

_____

_____

_____

_____

_____

CHAPTER TWO

Simply Opening
Your Doors Is
Not Enough

*"An expert is someone who knows some of the worst mistakes,
which can be made, in a very narrow field."*
—NIELS BOHR

FIFTY PERCENT OF SMALL BUSINESSES close after five short years.
And of all the hearing care practices (i.e. businesses) that *do*
make it five years or more, 90% of the owners are making
within 10% of what they would be making if they were an
employee somewhere else. THAT IS CRAZY! Think about
it. Who in their right mind would become a business owner
and do all the things required of a business owner just to
make nearly the same salary they could make with a regular
job? Yet it happens every day in small business, and audiology
is no exception.

Patients won't come to—or stay at—your practice unless
you give them a good reason to. If you research the numerous
businesses who are forced to close their doors every year, you
will be horrified. Simply building it and opening the doors
does *not* bring people through the door. Look at Sears or
JCPenny. Their existence did not bring people in—because

that's not enough in today's market. And if you believe that audiology can survive on the retail approach (e.g., free give-aways, coupons, BOGO, etc.), you are dead wrong.

According to the U.S. Small Business Administration, about half of all businesses make it to five years, and less than 33% make it to ten years. Even if you set these facts aside for a minute, you can look around your community and observe this statistic first-hand. Most likely you can name several businesses that closed in the last year or so. Actually, these places were likely not bad; they didn't lack a good concept, and the owners were just as passionate about their businesses as you are about yours.

So where did they go wrong? It was because of one of two reasons—perhaps even both. Reason 1: They thought that opening their doors was enough. Reason 2: They got into business for the wrong *reason*. I've come across many small business owners who told me that they started their own business because they were tired of working for someone else. Sorry to be the bearer of bad news, but getting into business to be your own boss is not a good enough reason to get into business.

Being the owner of an audiology practice means that you don't have just one boss, but rather hundreds of "bosses" (in the form of patients) who hold you accountable every day. These types of business owners soon realize they can't take a vacation without the entire operation shutting down. What most business owners end up with is a *job that they can't quit.* Combine this issue with the fact that many small business owners do little or no research into the marketplace prior to opening their doors, and you have a recipe for disaster, or at best, mediocrity. If they had done their due diligence, they may have found that there are nine other area businesses in the same category who are also struggling. This is simply not a smart way to go into a new business. But in fact, it's pretty close to the way most hearing care practice owners go into business today, the only difference being that hearing care professionals need a formal education and license to open a practice.

In the past, the audiology industry had the odds in their favor based upon statistics—the aging population, a robust economy, and a lack of licensed providers to service the demand. Then came the start of the Great Recession of 2008, and now, out of nowhere, over-the-counter hearing aids are on our doorstep.

We were immensely spoiled before the recession of 2008, just like other small business owners were. But now we have the newest assault, the OTC hearing aid assault. You may or may not remember when the American consumer had easy access to credit, often their home equity line. Back then, as a society, we spent more than we made, we didn't save, we went to restaurants too often, and we rarely thought about the "unlikely collapse" that would happen as home values rose. Then, like a smack in the face, things started to collapse, and today, everything is different. We are uncertain of the future, worried about the next collapse, and fearful of the big box stores, discount houses, and aggression of OTC

WHAT IS YOUR HOURLY RATE?

What are you worth? Seriously, when was the last time you calculated your value in dollars? How much money are your time, effort, blood, sweat, and tears worth? What are your nights and weekends worth? What is the cost of not spending enough time with your family and friends, not focusing on the things you truly love about life? Put bluntly, **if you are not receiving the income you deserve for all your time, why are you doing it?**

Too often I have to break the news to my clients that they are paying themselves at a rate equivalent to a high school fast food worker. In many cases, my clients would be better off (both financially and emotionally!) if they let me take over the business and pay them the salary they deserve. And I mean it when I say that. Several of my clients have taken me up on my offer to take over their practice, and they now work as part of my team. And as a result, they make a very nice steady paycheck and enjoy the freedom of working *in* their practice and not constantly working *on* their practice.

CALCULATE YOUR REAL HOURLY WAGE

Most private practice owners' take-home salary is within 10% of what they would make if they had a typical 9-to-5 audiology job. Yet owners work an astronomically more than the 40-hour-per-week audiologist. When you truly count all of the extra work and time that goes into running a practice to determine an actual hourly wage, my clients are shocked to learn that they are only paying themselves a mere pittance, and they don't have the cash flow to pay themselves anymore.

WHAT YOU SHOULD BE MAKING

Here is the simple formula that practice owner needs to know. **If your hourly wage and annual income aren't more than _triple_ what it would be as an employed audiologist, you are doing something wrong!**

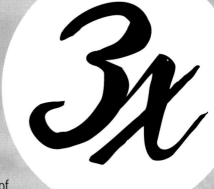

Yes, it takes work and dedication to get there, but that is what I do for practices that I work with. Our proven systems are able to provide the private practice owner with the tools and resources they need to succeed in every market.

And if you aren't making triple, you need to dig deep and understand why. Believe me, it is not because you have a big box retailer down the street from you selling low-cost widgets (I have two of them within a mile of my office!).

The tools and resources my team at AuDExperts have built can help you understand your worth and help you grow your practice to bring home that triple income you deserve.

hearing aid manufacturers. So what is the smart thing to do? Learn from past business failures and build a strong practice that will thrive into the future.

WARNING: I welcome OTC hearing aids with open arms. While this may come as a shock to you, and possibly offend you, I believe the more people in our society talk about hearing health care, the better.

Let's discuss another lie in business. We were always told that if we do good work, we will succeed. But that's not always true, and it's definitely *not guaranteed!* You could be the world's best hearing care professional, but being good is just one portion of a multifaceted business puzzle. You must be more than just a good hearing health care provider—you have to be *great* at what you do, and even greater at talking about it! In today's business world, you must be so amazing that people take notice and are willing to dodge all the other piranhas in the river just to get to your front door, to wait in line, and to pay full price for what you do for them. *Does this happen at your practice?* It does at mine.

If you find yourself asking—and I'm pretty sure you do—how to reach more people, the first thing you must understand is your market position. You need to know who you are, what you stand for, and who your "A" patient is. If you don't, you will quickly kill your practice or yourself trying to be all things to everyone and everything in your practice. This includes the patients who are impossible, under any circumstance, to work with—even if God himself was the hearing care professional! Clearly define your position in the market, and then *dominate it!* Articulate who you are looking for, and then draw those patients to you like a magnet. Yes, you can make yourself magnetic!

I'll give you a great example of this concept—Apple Inc. They clearly defined their position in the market. They create for a specific niche of people and not for others. What would happen if Apple changed who they are to fit in with everyone? What if they changed their products and service to be more like Microsoft or Google? Would they piss off their die-hard Mac fans? Yes. Would they ever satisfy Microsoft and Google followers? Definitely not.

Consider the famous quote, "Jack of all trades, master of none." This principle applies when you try to be all things to all patients. What you do end up being is nothing to no one. You must determine your *exact* position in the market, then you begin to attract the correct patients to your practice.

As another example, consider the luxury car market, and let's use Cadillac as our example. Cadillac has a fully defined position in the market on purpose. What would happen if Cadillac attempted to appease the same customers who were searching for a cheap, basic vehicle that simply got them where they needed to go? And on the other side of the coin, what if Nissan started building cars like Cadillac? This doesn't work. You need to understand this idea clearly. Neither position in the market is right or wrong, but each position is *exactly* right for each respective business. Both companies are true to their positions in the market. They have done their research and gone into detail to know and understand who their specific client is and how to serve them. Decisions are based upon their position in the market and staying true to serving their specific clientele.

Knowing that, let's stop and consider the audiology practices you know. Who do they think their ideal patient is? Everyone with hearing loss, right? Nearly all of my new coaching clients on their initial diagnostic phone call believe their market segment includes anyone with ears. Baloney! I could look at your profit and loss statement from last year and quickly tell you who your market sector is and determine who it should be. Hint: it's generally the top five to twenty percent of your patients who have paid you the overwhelming majority of your income. Are you familiar with the Pareto principle—the 80/20 rule? If not, now would be a good time to look it up. It has yet to fail me in any aspect of my business.

According to research by the Gartner Group, 80% of your future revenues will come from 20% of your existing patients. In my own practice, I have found this number to sometimes be as low as 5–10%. What about the bottom of your pyramid? Those are the patients that owe you money, won't do anything unless insurance pays for it, constantly complain about nearly everything, write negative reviews, and cause the burnout of so many of our peers. A friend of mine who is a university professor told me that when he first started, 5% of the trouble students took up nearly 95% of his time and energy. But then he changed his mindset, and now he focuses on the students who show up and do their job; he is there for those students whenever they need him. You need to do the same for the patients that matter the most, the ones who care the most, and the ones who love that you are their doctor or specialist.

Your best market segment is the top 20% of your practice that loves coming to see you, always has fun in the office, refers friends and family, pays without resistance or issue, and generally loves that you are their hearing care professional. If you can't determine within that segment the precise "hot buttons" that make this group act, or if you are a new practice that needs more patients, you can work backwards to get what you need.

Initially, **you must determine what sets you apart from others.** How are you different? How are you unique? Are you a category of one? What are the most frequent facets of you and your business that your patients compliment you on? Let's say you live in an area like I do with a senior population of 25,000, and there are 15 hearing care practices to choose from. Before you can even begin to differentiate, you must know how you are different, or how you *want* to be different. Why would a patient choose you over any other options in your area or market—including the option of doing absolutely nothing at all for their audiology needs?

Once you stake your claim in a specific segment of the market, then you will be in the best position to form the perfect strategy which will allow you to build your brand based upon the value you provide and your points of differentiation. If you think you can skip over this, or choose not to determine this first, you will not get far in practice. You will end up being just another practice in the market, and you will be driven to the lowest common denominator of selling hearing "widgets" based on price.

In my practice, I've gone to great lengths never to compete on price, and it has worked well for me and for my clients around the country. My best recommendation for you is to differentiate and charge accordingly. If you need a kick-start, try visiting luxury brands or experiences like Disney Parks or Jaguar, or just grab Dan Kennedy's book *No B.S. Price Strategy: The Ultimate No Holds Barred, Kick Butt, Take No Prisoners Guide to Profits, Power, and Prosperity.*

You might be the best practitioner in your state, the country, or even the world, but if you don't learn how to spread your message, market your skills, and get butts in the seats (or hire someone who will) you'll never get a chance to share your expertise with the world. Many businesses fail simply because they don't know how to market what they do. It's really very basic. If you've ever run an ad that focuses on a widget, practice name, location, phone number, address, or hours of operation, you are committing a huge marketing sin. Please promise me that moving forward you will *never ever have an ad that focuses on any of the above items.*

I often laugh when my newspaper representative calls me before running an ad to tell me, "You forgot your logo," or, "You forgot your address." These things do not matter. **The *message* you get across in the advertisement is what matters.** And it matters way more than your address. After all, if your message doesn't get across, then they don't really care what your logo looks like because they are never going to look at it. However, if your message *does* resonate, patients will seek you out.

For example, I have patients that drive from Salt Lake City to my practice in St. George (that is an 8-hour round-trip drive!). Why? Because of my message of value-added hearing health care that focuses on the patient and not the widget connected with them. *I have differentiated my practice.*

Marketing is not meant to be fun or recreational in nature. Stop behaving like the competition, and start holding your advertising accountable and tracking the return on investment. Your marketing budget should never be wasted by throwing money into the world to help brand who you are, where you are located, and when your office is open or closed. (Remember Chapter 1, "Quit Thinking It's About You!") Instead, start spending your marketing money moving potential patients through the buying lifecycle beginning with educating them on how you are different from others and how you can solve their problems better than any other practitioner in your community.

Please don't fret. You do not need to become a marketing expert overnight. However, all great leaders will either know how to take their practice to the next level or will get the assistance they need to make sure it gets done. In other words, if all this talk about marketing, market positioning, differentiation, and lifecycle marketing is making your head spin, then take the necessary steps to hire someone who is qualified and experienced to do it for you.

There are great doctors, audiologists, and hearing care professionals all over this country who are in poor locations, don't have a good team behind them, and have no systems in place for running a practice each day. The repercussions? Practices shutting down, selling out to large groups of retail clinics, and just plain giving up. Add into the mix an onslaught of OTC advertising in the coming years. With these and many other industry pressures, the profit margins we once enjoyed and the ready and willing patients will continue to dry up.

I'm sure you've heard it before, but the definition of insanity is doing the same thing over and over again but expecting a different result. Don't ever lose sight of the real facts in our industry—more people than ever are seniors. More than 10,000 people a day turn 65 years old. Eighty percent of people with hearing loss do not treat their hearing loss. And plenty of people pay lots of money for luxury cars when they are able to purchase a lower-cost car that will still get them from point A to point B. Trust me, our future in hearing health care is bright!

Bottom line—**you must effectively position your practice if you want to survive the coming years.** I highly recommend to all of my coaching clients, which in-

MOST SMALL BUSINESS BRANDING SUCKS *& here's how to fix it!*

I recently came across an article online from Sheena White in which she highlights what branding is REALLY all about (and FYI, it doesn't mention anything about a pretty logo!).

1 : GO ABOVE AND BEYOND ON YOUR PROMISES

The first piece of the puzzle is making a promise, keeping it, and then **going above and beyond to exceed expectations.**

2 : ALIGN YOURSELF WITH INFLUENCERS AND WELL-KNOWN BRAND AMBASSADORS

What do you do when you want to make your brand appeal to a wide range of people in a niche market? You **align yourself with someone who has the authority, recognition, and trust.**

3 : GREAT DESIGN IS NOW EXPECTED

Invest in great design. Remember, great design evokes strong emotions, and if you don't have a great design on everything that is out there, you are not going to stand out.

4 : CONSISTENCY RULES THE DAY

While great design can help get people excited, it's **consistency that creates trust.**

5 : GIVE YOUR BEST STUFF AWAY FOR FREE

Regardless of your business or industry, there's always a way you can give stuff away for free. And don't be lame and just give away a simple hearing test (BORING!). **Make your free stuff so good that people will be shocked you're not charging for it.**

you, the book *Positioning: The Battle for Your Mind* by Al
nd Jack Trout. Reading this book is going to reiterate rec-
ommendations of positioning and differentiation in your market. Just as a scientist diligently studies research, white papers,
and specialty pieces, you must review classic business literature,
case studies, and market research. These timeless concepts and
strategies will determine your success moving forward.

Long gone are the days when the hearing care professional
could graduate, open their clinic doors, and just watch patients
walk in the office day after day. Deciding to open a practice,
build an office, and open the door does *not* mean patients will
magically appear. There are more hearing care options today
than ever before, including large corporate chains, third-party
groups, big box stores, and discount houses—not to mention
OTC hearing aids. This causes mass consumer confusion, and
it's the new landscape of hearing healthcare. Welcome!

Are you ready to build a stronger foundation? If so,
then read on.

ACTION ITEMS WHAT WILL YOU DO NEXT?

_____

_____

_____

_____

_____

_____

_____

_____

_____

_____

_____

_____

_____

_____

_____

_____

_____

_____

_____

_____

_____

_____

_____

_____

_____

_____

_____

_____

_____

_____

_____

_____

CHAPTER THREE

Stop Selling.
You Suck at It!

"At the end of the day we are not selling, we are serving."
—DAVE RAMSEY

IT IS ESTIMATED THAT NEARLY 48,000,000 PEOPLE suffer with hearing loss, yet 40,000,000 (83%) do nothing about it. Even worse, in the hearing health care industry, only 35% of people who get tested by a hearing health care provider and have hearing loss actually begin treatment. So I say this as politely as possible—you suck at selling, so please, stop doing it!

If you are looking to settle for average and can tolerate nearly 65% of your efforts being wasted by people walking out the door, be my guest. Even better, send them to one of my practices or one of my clients' that is near your clinic because I know my providers, and the ones I coach will be happy to take care of your no-sale/not-helped patients. But then again, because you are reading this right now and looking for information on being more successful, I don't think that's what you want to do at all.

I want to see you through to the day when your practice starts treatment on 85–90% of new patients who visit your office for consultations. Can you really imagine your life achieving maximum impact and true wealth as the owner of your business with desirable assets? I can. Can you see yourself taking action towards this vision? I can. And it all begins with the most valuable asset in your practice.

What is the most valuable asset in your practice? Well, I can tell you, it is not your building. It is not your equipment, your staff, or your accounts receivable. Nope. **Your most valuable asset is your database.** There are two groups within your database, and each patient falls into one of these two categories:

1. The patient who has invested in hearing health care at your office.
2. The patient who has raised his or her hand to let you know that they need help with their hearing impairment, but they are too nervous or "just not ready" to commit to hearing health care.

Let me ask you, and I really want you to think about this, can you list at least ten things that you did last month to purposefully strengthen the relationship that you have with your patient list? Did you have a patient appreciation event? (And if so, did you have more than 100 patients attend?) Did you send birthday cards? Did you send every patient in your database an e-mail about the new research published in *The*

Lancet in July of 2017 indicating that treating hearing loss is the single most effective means of preventing dementia? I did each one of these things in my practice—and many more.

I'm curious, did you just read that last paragraph and say, "That is too much for my patients," or, "My patients would get upset if I contacted them that often"? Well, my response is, *no,* it's not too much; and I know it's not too much because less than 2% of my 10,000+ patients have opted out of my nurture campaigns. Or perhaps you are asking yourself, "How could I possibly add all of those things on my *to-do* list?" Well, that's easy. I can help you figure out how to do all of these things with ease and find you the right DFY (Done For You) in our industry.

Hmm, you haven't put in much effort to build a relationship with them? Well, that's definitely a problem. You must make your patient list a priority if you want to have a successful practice. Consider Walt Disney again. The people who visit his theme parks do not sit around talking about the mechanics of each ride or the specific features of the hotel beds, and they don't wax poetic about the breakfast buffet. Instead, they share extensive stories about their experiences with Disney and how their relationship with Disney from a young age and the magic of Disney have kept them coming back over the years.

Your practice is no different than this. Your patients are not going to tell their friends and family stories about the newest instruments you use or the plaques hanging on your wall. They will, though, rave about the experience and relationship they have with you—if you get it right.

If you have gone to any of my events, or if you have seen me on stage in front of thousands of audiology professionals just like you, then you have heard me say that you could repossess my buildings or burn them to the ground, ship my entire staff to Mars, throw all of my equipment in the river, and if you simply give me six months and my patient list, and I would rebuild it all back. That's not a lie nor an exaggeration. Why? Because I have learned and understand that the most valuable asset in my practices is my relationship with my patient list. Believe it or not, everything else can be replaced. The relationship you have with your patient list is golden, and it needs to be treated as such for it to thrive.

So the question again is **what are you doing this month to build a relationship with your patients?** If you don't know the answer, you have definite room for improvement. You need to address this issue *now* before it is too late. Start today. Form a plan, set new goals, and make your focus building a great relationship with your patients. If you don't take the time to do this, your patients will more than likely leave in search of someone who will. And there's a chance one of my clients who gets this right is already in your area patiently waiting.

Did you realize that the average clinic owner—approximately 85% percent of them—spends between 5–10% of their revenue per year promoting and marketing their practices? Let's ponder that for a moment. That's pocket change. It's just not enough to really make an actual impression. And it's unquestionably not enough to gain much market share or generate a steady message for your relationship with your patient list.

Extensive research confirms that about 15% of practice owners are really positive about their future in business. Only 15%. That, unfortunately, does not surprise me at all. So who are the 15% that are truly optimistic? They are the same owners who spend more than 15% a year endorsing their practices. They are the ones who are getting the relationship right, and they understand *why* they are in business, *who* they are in business to serve, and *how* to control the relationship they have with the patient list. Those are the 15%.

They are optimistic because they are explicitly capitalizing on new patient acquisition, fostering patient relationships, following up with those who are "not sure," and constructing systems for employees to produce exceptional, unique, and memorable experiences for patients and staff. They are the practice owners who pay their teams at least 10% more than what they ask for because they deserve every penny of it (not because of the letters after their names). They are the hearing care professionals who are optimistic about their future in business. And quite frankly, they should be because they've got it right.

Where do you fall in this group? Do you want to quit making the same mistakes over and over again? Are you ready to make things happen? *Now* is the time to get serious and take real action on the road to results that will make your practice stand out and become more successful.

You must begin to make this change immediately. And if you aren't serious about it, you will *not* see substantial changes in your business. The goal of reading this book is to make significant change and achieve massive growth. But you *must* take the necessary action *now* to make these things transpire.

The must-implement actions you will now become acquainted with are relationship building, marketing, and employee training. Doing this will ensure that you are forming a patient experience like no one else. As I said previously, you don't have to be an expert at this. You and all of your staff can learn it. It is basically just a matter of taking initiative and getting it started. Buying this book was your first step and a great decision. It means that you have already begun the process. You are now entering the select class of the top 15% of practice owners who "get it" and comprehend that the future of our audiology profession must be totally restructured if we want to attain our personal and financial goals while still upholding the high-quality medical treatment of hearing loss.

I'm frequently stunned at the absence of action most business owners have taken with regard to communication skills, marketing, business management, and treatment plan presentations. Patients come to us with a fear of the doctor, fear that it means they are getting old and going deaf, fear of expensive treatment and many other unknowns. Unfortunately, very few hearing care professionals have researched these fears in depth, and even fewer have a strategy which translates into results.

My teachings have been known to take treatment coordinators from an average of 30–50% treatment rate to consistently above 85% (with many specialists above 90%). The skills we all now have in common are not magic. These skills do not require you to be remarkably captivating. You don't have to "sell" anything. All you need to do is build trust, continually act in your patients' best interests, present a treatment plan that will work best for every patient as an individual, and demonstrate self-confidence to the patient and family members as their trusted specialist and advisor. That's all. When meeting with new hearing care patients, this will only take about five to seven minutes of your initial consultation. Yup, that's all.

Ill-advisedly, a lot of professional talk way too much, give too much technical detail about the 'widget,' and then walk out of the room hoping that the treatment coordinator closes the case. This is the wrong process. You may be thinking that you are not guilty of this. If that is the case, then I challenge you to record your treatment presentations for one week, review them with your treatment coordinator, and see if you are doing this 100% correct. Clue: if you do not begin treatment on 90% or more of the cases you are recording, then there is room for improvement.

IF DISNEY RAN YOUR AUDIOLOGY PRACTICE...

A while back, I was bowling with a colleague, and he said to me, "You know, patient satisfaction drives revenue." This thought has never left my mind.

However, while I agree with his sentiment, I have since come to realize patients are really looking for an *experience*, not just satisfaction. Thus, I believe more in the motto, **"Patient *experience* drives revenue."**

Think about it. *Satisfaction* is not the same as *experience*. For many years major health care systems have been trying to improve patient satisfaction. By all accounts, satisfaction in health care has gone up in recent decades because Sally the clinician can meet all of her clinical goals and all of her expectations. But, what hasn't changed, is the public's perception of health care, and **when patients are asked to rate their *experience*, the results are very different.**

Disney is not looking for you to be satisfied with your time at their parks and hotels. **They are looking for you to have a *magical experience*.** What does that mean? Think about a non-Disney park you have been to with your family, and I would bet that the experience and memories cannot compare to your time at Disney. And trust me, the Disney "experience" is not something that happens by chance (e.g., you just "happened" to get a nice waiter or ride engineer). No, the Disney experience is a well thought-out process intentionally designed to "wow" you.

WHAT ARE YOU DOING TO "WOW" YOUR PATIENTS EVERY DAY?

What do you send to prospective patients? At my practices, we send the #1 Amazon best-selling book, *Stop Living In Isolation*, that is written by the only neuroscientist and clinical audiologist in our field and designed to educate and prepare your patients for their experience in your office. We also include a welcome DVD, a letter, and more.

Let's think about what you are doing for patients after they leave your office and have decided to invest in you for their hearing health care. How do you "wow" each patient you treat? Do you send a hand-written card to every patient? Does your thank-you packet include another copy of the book to give to a friend, a $50 gift card to a local restaurant, and other fun items that enhance their experience?

The experience you want your patients to have must be obvious in everything you do. Your website, your phones team, your patient care coordinators, your doctors, and even you. Every patient must know that you are in this for them, that you care about every aspect of their experience with you.

So why does the patient's experience matter? My simple answer is this. Over the last two weeks, 78% of new patients seen at my practice were from direct patient referrals! Imagine if your practice spent as much money on caring about your current patients as it does trying to get *new* patients in the door? What if your practice established a strong, experience-based relationship and 8 (or more) out of every 10 new patients that walked through your doors said "Yes" to treatment (i.e. an 80% conversion rate)?

What if that experience-based relationship with every patient resulted in your patients trusting your recommendation to upgrade their treatment when necessary, with no questions asked—and you no longer had to hear, "I just bought these widgets three years ago. I'm not spending more money!

What would a boost of 50% more patients investing in treatment every three to four years do for your bottom line while at the same time your in-house referrals were also increasing and you had an 80% conversion rate? Pretty mind-blowing!

In my practice and the practices I work with around the country, this is the reality of how their practice operates and why they grow at numbers our industry has never seen before.

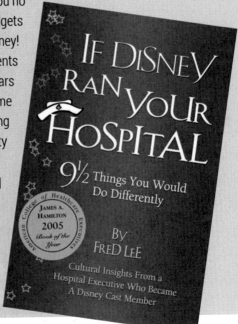

If you haven't done so, I strongly recommend you read Fred Lee's *If Disney Ran Your Hospital: 9 1/2 Things You Would Do Differently.*

Some of the most successful businesses in the world videotape and secretly shop their sites all the time. When was the last time you sent a secret patient to your practice? Would you want to see the results, or would you be too fearful of what you might discover? And my favorite—are you afraid that your employees would be mad at you for secret shopping them? Ha! As if they have any right to tell you, the business owner, the person that everything mentally and financially falls upon, "Don't you ever secret shop me!" Guess what—it's not about them either. (Make sure they read Chapter 1!)

In my coaching program, audiologists and specialists around the globe are now pledging to give this tactic a try in their businesses at least once or twice a year. I have to tell you that I have been doing this for a long time at my locations, and every time I learn something new. You will learn how long your patients wait in the reception area—if you have a reception area. You will learn how it feels to be a new patient in your practice. You will learn how you are greeted at the door. What does the office look like from the patient's perspective? You will learn how it sounds, feels and smells in the reception area.

You may think that this is going a little too far and sounds a little harsh. But take a look at some of the most widely successful businesses such as the Ritz-Carlton. A friend and trusted advisor in the orthodontics industry has actual scent machines in his office, and his staff bakes fresh cookies in house every day (and who doesn't love the smell of fresh baked cookies?). He uses the same method as the Ritz-Carlton, and they both know exactly what their ultimate customer experience really looks like.

Your business's transformation needs to start with a candid evaluation of the realities in your practice. If you want to start knowing, with *certainty*, how much money you will make tomorrow, next week, or next month, I can tell you with equal certainty that this is a step you must take. If you disagree, I reassure you that if you schedule a secret mystery patient to visit your practice, you will find something to improve upon. I take this seriously and do it faithfully. Without performing this, how can we *really* know what is going on in our practices.

ACTION ITEMS WHAT WILL YOU DO NEXT?

_____

_____

_____

_____

_____

_____

_____

_____

_____

_____

_____

_____

_____

_____

_____

_____

_____

_____

_____

_____

_____

_____

_____

_____

_____

_____

_____

_____

_____

_____

_____

_____

_____

_____

CHAPTER FOUR

You're a Doctor.
Whoopdee-Freakin'
Doo!

"Arrogance is a creature. It does not have senses.
It has only a sharp tongue and the pointing finger."
—TOBA BETA

READ THIS SENTENCE AND ENGRAIN IT into your mind: ***You are***
not entitled to anything. The worst thing you can do is
think that the industry, or your credentials, somehow owes
you something.

This may sound harsh because I know that you have
worked hard, but simply graduating from audiology school
and earning the title "doctor," or becoming board-certified,
does not in any way put you in a special category of entitle-
ment. This truth may deflate you a bit, but it is the truth in
the working world.

I did the same thing as you. I went to business school and
beyond and earned an MBA. However, earning that title never
meant that I was entitled to anything. Nothing will ever be handed to you. Not even close! Accept that fact now and move on.

Get rid of the notion that you will come to the office,
work on ears and auditory systems, and leave everything else

on the back burner while you drive home at 4:30. Because this recipe is meant for an exceptionally average practitioner with an average number of patients, average staff productivity, average income, and an average number of referrals. Successful audiology practice owners realize this little secret, the one that no one in school shared with you.

If it were that simple, there would be no need to write (or read) this book. The most successful individuals in any field reach their highest level of achievement through plain old blood, sweat, and tears. In an exposé of Marissa Mayer years back (who until recently was one of the highest-paid CEOs in Silicon Valley), when asked how she rose to the helm at Yahoo! at such a young age, she responded, "I like to work." Boom!

No one in a position of power, prestige, or high income got where they are simply because of their title or due to good genes, luck, or any other excuse that unsuccessful people use to relieve themselves of the hard work and results achieved by the top 1% in any field. Harsh, but true. It's easier to accept an alibi for your lack of results in life than to risk and fail. Every entrepreneur and top 1% audiology practice owner achieved their position through risk, failure, determination, hard work, blood, sweat, and tears. Don't think it will be any different for you.

Let's look at a few more famous people who had to take action to get where they are today:

ROHAN OZA

Oza is without a doubt, one of the most successful entrepreneurs in marketing in the United States. Oza has accumulated millions due to his success in making food and beverage products into brands that people around the world recognize, including Vita Coco, Vitaminwater, and Pop Chips. Before that, he helped to fix and turn around the success and fortune of Powerade and Sprite by boosting revenue via his innovative brand endorsements. But Oza did not have it all handed to him on a silver platter. He began his career in manufacturing for the brand M&M. He has come a long way by never giving up and using his creativity to become the businessman he is today.

JUDD APATOW

Famous for his comedy writing and producing, he tops the lists on being one of the smartest people in Hollywood. And rightfully so. This man didn't just cash in some luck to get where he is. He stayed up late at night to write and rewrite scripts by hand while watching Saturday Night Live. Sure, he could have taken the night off, relaxed, and just laughed with a beer in his hand. But that wasn't enough for him. He wanted to know what it felt like as a young writer to see exceptional comedic writing flow effortlessly from his pen, so he put in the long hours and the extreme measures that others in his field avoided by transcribing his words of Saturday Night Live by hand, over and over again. His hard work and determination helped push him to the top of his industry. Self-sacrifice. Decisive action in pursuit of his goals. He did not wait for an easy button to appear. That reminds me of an old Far Side cartoon with two hungry vultures waiting for their next meal. The caption read: "Screw this. Let's go kill something." When will you stop waiting around for everything to go your way without devoting massive effort? It's simply not easy.

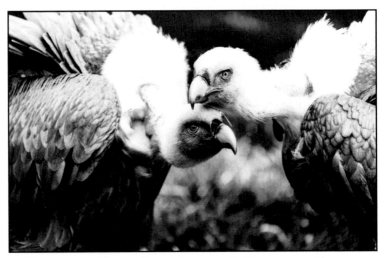

Screw this. Let's go kill something.

RICHARD BRANSON

Did you know that Richard Branson dropped out of school at the age of 16 and suffered from dyslexia? Yet he immediately started a youth-culture magazine

YOU'RE A DOCTOR. WHOOPDEE-FREAKIN' DOO! 83

called *Student*. The publication, run by students, for students, sold $8,000 worth of advertising in its first edition—at the age of 16! Of course, his entrepreneurial quests didn't end there. He went on to create Virgin Records. He then expanded into other sectors and became a billionaire. He is also well known for his adventurous spirit and sporting achievements, including crossing oceans in a hot air balloon. But nothing was handed to Branson. His massive achievements were all due to his own drive, motivation, hard work, and creativity. Did he have losses? Yes! But, his desire for success made him put those losses aside and move on.

HENRY FORD

One of America's leading entrepreneurs, Ford developed and transformed assembly-line modes of production for the automobile. Today, he is credited with helping to shape America's economy during our weak early years and will always be considered one of America's great leading businessmen. Aside from creating the great Model T, the first car to be reasonably priced for most Americans, he launched the first assembly line for mass production of the automobile. This system reduced the amount of time it took to build a car from 12 hours to 2.5 hours, which in turn lowered the cost even further. In 1914, Ford announced the $5 an hour wage, which was more than double what employees were formerly making for the most part, as a way of keeping the best workers devoted to his company. But even better than all of that, Ford became notorious for his groundbreaking vision: the production of a low-priced automobile completed by skilled employees who earned solid wages.

THOMAS EDISON

When you think of Thomas Edison, you probably think of a really successful guy who had a lot of skill and intuition. And you would be right. But what you may not realize is that he had many more failures than he had successes; he just didn't focus on those failures. He paid more attention to the success and kept on going. Failed attempts were either pushed aside or used as learning experiences so he could go on to something more successful. When asked about his many unsuccessful attempts at developing the lightbulb, he said, "I didn't invent the lightbulb, but instead found 10,000 ways *not* to invent the lightbulb."

MICHAEL JORDAN

You know he was good, but that doesn't mean Jordan was born that way. Rather, he put in more effort training and becoming the best of the best than most people could imagine. While there are trainers and specialists that work with basketball teams, he went above and beyond. Michael went outside the team and hired his own coaches and did his own training regimens. He had dedication to personal improvement when other players simply wouldn't put in the same amount of time. If you asked him to retell the stories of last-second, game-winning shots, he would quickly redirect the conversation to all of the times he had the opportunity to win the game but failed. Imagine that. The greatest basketball player on earth and he quickly focused on his relatively infinitesimal number of failures. He was always focused on doing better and was quick to recognize that doing better meant hard work—not luck, not genes, not resting on prior successes.

Many non-achievers find it easy to simply say that people are successful because it was handed to them, or even because they were born with "that special something." By using these excuses, instead of being inspired, it becomes easier to forget about their own lack thereof. Why do people do this? Because if they actually believed that we all have the ability to achieve superstar status, they would have to ask themselves why they have not yet achieved all they desire. And then they would have to admit that what they are doing is wrong.

In other words, by being inspired and admitting your faults, you will know it's time to take massive action and make things happen.

At times we just find it easier to make do with the excuses we have built up in our heads. We have a habit of complaining about our patient relationships, but we do nothing to foster those relationships. Some complain that their staff isn't working hard to get referrals, yet they do nothing to train, encourage, and praise the results when they do. If you are reading this right now, then it is imperative that you improve referral communication and strengthen referral sources. It is also imperative that you decide today, once and for all, to abandon the excuses in your head forever. When we complain about our position when it comes to referrals—or anything else really—we are really making a statement about our own engagement and responsibility to our practices. You cannot complain on the one hand without criticizing yourself on the other.

The choice is yours. Will you focus on building referral relationships and teaching your team to do the same? If you don't know how many patients will call your office tomorrow, next week, or next month with near-certainty, you need to pay attention and do the work to fix the problem. Unfortunately, we weren't taught how to manage and leverage these essential success strategies while earning the letters after our names. For those of you with serious interest, resources are available (including the ones presented here) to help catapult your practice into the position necessary to explode your success for the lifetime of your practice. The solutions in this book may not always be easy, but they are tested and proven, not only in our field, but throughout the business world in general. You do not need to be remarkably charismatic to apply any of these strategies, nor do you have to turn your employees into annoying salesmen to function in the top 1% of audiology practices. You only need to follow simple directions and formulas, take responsibility, and get started. Graduating from audiology school, or becoming board-certified, was really just the beginning.

ACTION ITEMS WHAT WILL YOU DO NEXT?

_____

_____

_____

_____

_____

_____

_____

_____

_____

_____

_____

_____

_____

_____

_____

CHAPTER FIVE

Practice Owners Often Retire Poor

"Wealth is the progressive realization of worthy goals."
—DEEPAK CHOPRA

THE TITLE OF THIS CHAPTER MAY BE SHOCKING TO YOU, and it should be. I'm pretty sure you did not fight your way through audiology school, graduate with mountains of debt, or spend years becoming board-certified in a new profession, only to retire poor. But that is the reality for a lot of hearing care professionals. There are too many hearing care professionals that make this crucial mistake. But this is completely avoidable if you take the appropriate action.

So how exactly does this happen? You spend your days, nights, and weekends working hard in your practice and making a decent salary only to walk away in the end with nothing. Well, let me tell you how it happens for the majority. It largely comes down to you and what you do *during* your career.

What you do presently and in future years is going to be the difference between whether you retire poor or not, and whether you get to continue living the lifestyle you deserve or not. It basically comes down to you and the decisions you make.

Most clinic owners, approximately 80%, will not retire with the same amount of retirement income as they had when they were actively practicing. Shame on us. We can do so much better than that.

Lifestyle choices while in practice are one thing, but it's a very different story to allow a gross underestimation of the level of revenue you need, and how to invest, when to buy a building versus lease one, and how to leverage your number one business expense—payroll—into an army of advocates that can build your retirement at the same time they are building their own through a company-sponsored retirement plan.

When you ponder the fact that 80% of us will retire with less income than we now enjoy, it would be crazy to continue on the way that you are. This is called willful ignorance. But ignorance is *not* bliss.

Private practice owners are leaving too much money on the table every day, week, month and year they are in practice—and a whole lot of money behind once they finally retire. You have a choice to make. *You* do not have to be willfully ignorant. *You* can choose right here and right now to learn everything you can and put it all into action so that you are not one of the those who retires poor.

You see, it's just not enough to finish audiology school, become a doctor or board-certified professional, and believe that you can sail through your career. It simply does not hap-

HIGH INCOME VS HIGH NET WORTH

BUILDING WEALTH REQUIRES A STRATEGIC SHIFT IN MINDSET.

The "traditional" retirement model requires stockpiling mountains of cash. Financial advisors often advise stockpiling 2 to 4 million dollars or more.

The truly wealthy often don't earn more than their less wealthy peers—they just view that income differently and make their dollars work harder for them.

When I asked my peers how they are securing their future, their answers are scary:

"Traditional investments with 2% returns..."

Truckloads of cash dumped into the stock market with set-it-and-forget-it strategies. Or even worse—handing money to a stranger in a suit and hoping they can survive the stock market's roller coaster ride.

How much money you need to retire depends on how well that money works for you.

Calculate How Hard Your Money Is Working For You.

www.FreedomFounders.com/calculator

pen that way for the most successful individuals in any field, and it will not happen that way for you. You will never sail through your career successfully if you sweep the hard decisions under the rug and neglect the path less traveled—never. You will retire poor.

You must take full responsibility in running your practice successfully. You want your practice to run successfully, efficiently, and to your benefit. In doing this, you must be willing to leave ignorance behind. You must be willing to invest in yourself, your career, and importantly, in the information and strategies you need to assist you in realizing the level of success you dreamed of when you first applied to audiology school and opened the doors to your practice. I made that commitment a long time ago, and it has paid off greatly.

Now having read this, are you ready and willing to make that commitment for yourself, for the success of your practice, so that you can retire maintaining the lifestyle and legacy you want and dream of? Do you want to learn and comprehend what acquisition costs are, how much you spend on each prospect in your marketing and advertising, what type of return on investment each employee is earning for your business, and how to leverage every single dollar of income in your business so that your children can go to the kind of school they desire, so that your employees can retire comfortably just like you, so that your community, church, or synagogue can benefit from your generosity? You can answer these questions, and you can put the knowledge you gain into immediate action.

Don't let your hard-earned career rely on ignorance. You spent years going to school and developing the skills to practice your craft. Don't let that hard work or money be wasted by willfully ignoring the key strategies that can allow your talents to soar to newer and better heights.

The highest producers in any field are paid more for who they *are* as opposed to what they *do*. This is the single most important awareness you must recognize before you happily take the road less traveled. It will be the difference between having a run-of-the-mill practice and one that is extremely successful. It is going to be the difference between retiring poor or relishing in a larger-than-life retirement by leaving a legacy for you and your family.

You hold all the cards to make the difference. As the saying goes, you can lead a horse to water, but you can't make it drink. I can tell you what you need to learn and how specific things will power your practice results, but I cannot force you to *apply* those philosophies once you commit to learning them. Only *you* can take the decisive action in your practice.

It all comes down to you, the decisions you make, and what you desire for your future, both during your career and in retirement. Put yourself under a concentrated self-assessment, and then finally make the decisions that will help get you where you desire to be. And if you aren't aware of some of the best classic business literature available at the secret place

not often visited by hearing care professionals after gradua-
tion (called the library), I have included a few below for your
reference. And if you decide to read and apply the principles
contained within, well then, I've also saved you at least one
year's tuition in obtaining your MBA. You're welcome!

REQUIRED BUSINESS READING

The Innovator's Dilemma. Christensen, Clayton. New York: Harper

The Effective Executive. Drucker, Peter. New York: Harper Collins

The E-Myth Revisited. Gerber, Michael. New York: Harper Collins

Emotional Intelligence. Goleman, Daniel. New York: Bantam

Marketing Myopia. Levitt, Ted. Boston: Harvard Business Press

Competitive Strategy. Porter, Michael. New York: Free Press

ACTION ITEMS WHAT WILL YOU DO NEXT?

_____

_____

_____

_____

_____

_____

_____

_____

_____

_____

_____

_____

_____

_____

_____

_____

_____

_____

_____

_____

_____

_____

_____

_____

_____

_____

_____

_____

_____

_____

_____

_____

_____

_____

CHAPTER SIX

Patients Simply Don't Care About Your New Equipment

"I'd rather regret the things I've done than regret the things I haven't done."
—LUCILLE BALL

WITHOUT A DOUBT, YOU ARE EXCITED about the latest tool you purchased for your business. You are also very excited about a new continuing education course you are going to attend. Honesty, though, that stuff just does not mean anything to your patients—and it actually bores them. Disappointing, yes. But consider when the shoe is on the other foot. Do you want to sit around and hear all about the new gadget that your plumber just purchased when he comes out to fix your toilet? I'm going to venture a guess—no. Like everything else in life, there are a few exceptions to every rule, but most people pretty much tend not to care about such things.

However, there is something that entices your patients about the latest gadgets you purchased or the recent CE courses you attended, but only if it benefits *them*, not you. This goes all the way back to the first principle discussed in this guide. It's not about *you*. It's about *them*.

In other words, if you are not able to tell your patients in layman's terms how the latest and greatest thing is going to benefit them, their life, and the lives of their family and loved ones, then don't even mention it to them. Doing so will more than likely do nothing but bore them, perhaps even irritate them. Your time—and theirs—can be better spent. On the other hand, if it is something that *will* benefit them, by all means, tell them! Just leave aside the info about the device that you find interesting as a professional. Instead, tell them what it means for *them*. They will understand, relate to it, and appreciate it in the long run.

Another big news flash. Patients who come into your office, or who are at home looking at your website and wondering if they should make an appointment with you, also don't care about your specific association with any "occlusion camps." You might mention you studied "here" and you studied "there," but they more than likely have never even heard of these places, and they really don't care. It means absolutely nothing to them. They won't be impressed merely because you take a lot of continuing education. They already assume that you, as a professional, take a lot of continuing education. Again, what they truly care about is how this is going to benefit *them*.

If you spent $50,000 and months of your life studying "here" and "there" and you feel that it will benefit your patient, by all means, talk about it, but again, talk about it in layman's terms, and describe how your advanced training actually benefits them. Don't just show and brag; *prove*. Outside of that conversation, your voice sounds like the Charlie Brown's teacher ("wah, wah, wah, wah") and does nothing to help the patient—or your treatment rate for that matter. However, getting clear explanations in plain terms about how your training helps make their life easier will make them feel good about making the decision to choose your treatment over the competition. But keep it short and simple.

My favorite example of this is looking at the "About Us" page on different hearing health care practice websites. Sorry to break it to you, but warm and fuzzy bios don't attract patients to you. Turn the page to see an example of a bio I found on a website, and then I'll present you with an example of what it *should* say to actually motivate a patient to pick up the phone, book an appointment, and trust you with their hearing health care.

THE 'ABOUT US' PAGE ON 99% OF AUDIOLOGY WEBSITES

Our number one top priority is providing our patients with a comfortable, welcoming environment every time they visit the office. We know that treating your hearing loss can be a lengthy and stressful process. Dr. FuzzyBear will always provide you with many treatment options and work closely with you to create a personalized treatment plan that will fit both your lifestyle and budget.

Dr. FuzzyBear has been delivering outstanding Audiology care since XXXX. After receiving his Bachelor of Science degree from Some University, he then received his Doctorate of Audiology from Some Other University. A Fellow of the American Academy of Audiology, Dr. FuzzyBear maintains his state license and certificate of clinical competency with the American Speech-Language and Hearing Association.

When he is not at the office, Dr. FuzzyBear volunteers his time and talents to XYZ Charity and the National Order of Elks.

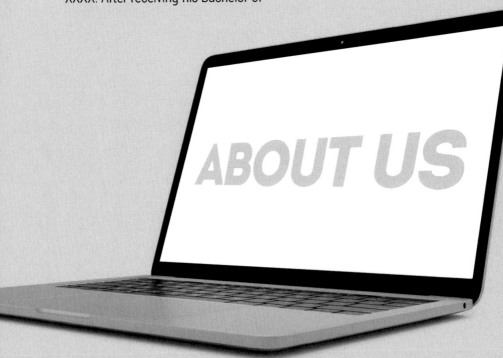

THE 'ABOUT US' PAGE ON THE LEADING 1% OF AUDIOLOGY WEBSITES

Dr. Authority is a nationally recognized speaker, teacher, author, and hearing care specialist. Since founding the Hearing Care Center in 2010, hundreds of audiologists have traveled to visit the practice from across the country to learn from Dr. Authority's vision to change lives, advance the profession, and support his community. Together, he and his hearing health care team and students treat hundreds of thousands of patients throughout North America each year.

Dr. Authority is part of a team that creates numerous professional monthly newsletters and is the Director of the Healthy Hearing Foundation. His practices have personally transformed the lives of over 11,000 patients right here in Somewhere County, and he has helped more people through his efforts with the nonprofit Healthy Hearing Foundation.

The author of an Amazon best-selling patient-based book, Stop Living in Isolation, Dr. Authority has been invited to speak throughout the world. He has been featured on FOX, iHEART Radio, and the Somewhere County Gazette. Dr. Authority and his practice have been voted the prestigious Best in Somewhere County for six years in a row.

His hearing care providers and staff have worked with the prestigious Disney Institute and Ritz-Carlton to bring the same 'wow' experience to the patients in our community. When asked what makes his practice different, Dr. Authority quickly replied with a warm smile, "It's our people, our culture, and our commitment to do whatever it takes to serve the best interest of our patients and their families." He continued, "Even if it means referring them to a cheaper option in town," or to his nonprofit foundation when patients are unable to afford treatment at Dr. Authority's facility.

Dr. Authority's offices at last count have over 15,000 satisfied patients, traveling from cities far away to be treated by one of Dr. Authority's certified hearing care specialists.

I hope you will agree the differences in these two examples are obvious!

Remember, it's not about you and how much you care. It's about them. And they want to know how you and everything in your practice will benefit them.

Not only will your patients not remember your gadgets and tools, but they also won't remember where you studied or the latest class you took. There is one thing they will remember though—how you made them *feel*.

How you and your staff make each and every patient feel is going to stick with them forever. It is, plain and simple, a feeling that will come about every single time they think about you and your office. And that feeling will arise every time they have a problem or every time they hear their grandchild at the school play. They will always remember how you made them feel.

Because people are going to remember, very clearly, how you made them feel, it is extremely important to **give them an excellent experience and treatment every time they are in your office.** This is a crucial element in your story if you want those same people to continue feeling warm and fuzzy about you 10 or even 20 years from now. But don't stop there.

If you provide excellent quality treatment but cannot communicate effectively to the patient, then why would they follow your advice? Show them how they can benefit from the options in your practice, and consistently thank them for choosing you to manage their hearing health care while making them feel good.

Another bottom line. Treat your patients well, build lasting relationships with them, provide an excellent experience, and you will create a loyal following who will send you referrals on a regular basis. Your patients will remember how you made them feel when their friend says, "I think I'm starting to have difficulty hearing. Do you have any advice?" Whether people are happy with their hearing care professional or not, they love to share their experiences with others. What you want to do is make sure that they are sharing positive information with their friends and family.

And you absolutely *do* have control over this.

I repeat, your control over referrals to your practice boils down to how well you treat your patients, each and every one of them, each and every visit. They are all valuable. Remember that they are the most important asset in your office.

Your emphasis on an excellent experience must come from everyone in your office, not just you. It is vital to have the correct employee in each position within your practice and that all employees are on board with your mission of providing the best possible hearing health care. It is imperative that you train your staff with effective and patient-focused scripting so that they will be able to successfully communicate everything you are doing that is going to benefit the patient.

Take my word, as soon as you begin getting this right, you will notice your practice elevating to a new level of suc-

WHY IS THE RITZ-CARLTON SO SUCCESSFUL?

Because your experience at their hotel has a significant impact on your life. Check out their website. They aren't talking about a special tool or new bed that will impress you. Instead, they use key phrases like "creating memories." The M.O. of the Ritz-Carlton is "Ladies and gentleman serving ladies and gentleman." If you don't understand what this means, go to a Ritz-Carlton and tell the lifeguard that your room was dirty, and just wait and see what happens!

Each Ritz-Carlton employee has a budget of up to $2,000 to enhance a guest's experience—not per incident, or per day, or per anything. Simply put, if an employee believes that they can enhance the experience of a guest, they have free rein to spend up to $2,000 to do so, without requiring approval from a manager. There are many stories of employees going above and beyond to enhance a guest's experience, but my personal favorite was about helping a handicapped woman get down to the beach. The story goes like this.

A waiter overheard a couple speaking together at dinner. The wife, who was in a wheelchair, was remarking to her husband how she was disappointed that she was unable to make it down to the beach (which required climbing stairs to get to). This gave the waiter an idea. When the couple showed up to dinner the next night, the waiter greeted them and informed the couple that he had a special table set aside for them. Overnight, the waiter had hired a team to come in and build a temporary ramp down to the beach. He had also set up a tent and a table directly on the beach to serve the couple dinner, and his manager only found out what he'd done after the dinner was done.

The couple didn't care how it got done; they didn't care what tools were used to build the ramp or what courses the handyman took to build the ramp. **All that mattered to them was that their lives were forever changed**, for the better, by the kindness of a waiter at a Ritz-Carlton Hotel.

What does your practice do to meaningfully impact the life of every patient (in addition to treating their hearing loss)?

cess. Are you ready to make this commitment? Take this chapter of information and put it into immediate action. Your patients will walk out your door feeling amazing with an enthusiastic attitude about your practice. This will quickly build your reputation and earn you many more word-of-mouth referrals. Take note, though. Do not think for a second that you can train your staff just once in this area. **You must provide constant, never-ending training.** It's the hallmark of the most successful companies in the world. People want to find a great company with highly trained employees on a mission to deliver exceptional service to the customer without fail. How?

Start with a monthly team exercise. Put aside a little bit of time every month to arrange your calendar for upcoming team trainings. Make them into a workshop, not a lecture, and definitely not just another meeting. (One of my favorite signs I have hanging on my door says, "I just left another meeting that should have been an e-mail.") This is a great time to ask your staff questions, get input, and discover as a team how you can better serve your patients. Following are a few sample themes you can utilize at your next team workshop training. The sooner you get started on these, the better.

■   What three products or services in our office do we provide at an incomparable level of quality, but nobody even knows we do it? How can we better present these services to our patients so that everyone knows exactly how they can benefit from such a product or service.

'hat products or services have our patients or our referring doctors demanded of us, even though we have not aggressively promoted them in our practice newsletter or on our website? Have we taken the time to survey our other patients to see if these products or services might interest them as well?

■ What are the top three reasons why our patients might ask us to start actively educating everyone in the practice about these products or services?

ACTION ITEMS WHAT WILL YOU DO NEXT?

_____

_____

_____

_____

_____

_____

_____

_____

_____

_____

_____

_____

_____

_____

_____

_____

CHAPTER SEVEN

You are an Entrepreneur. Step up, or Get Out of the Way!

"Courage is resistance to fear,
mastery of fear, not absence of fear."
—MARK TWAIN

YOU SPENT YEARS TO EARN THOSE CREDENTIALS, hard years to learn how to do what you do, and here I am telling you that you need to step up, or get out of the way—maybe even find something else to do with your life. Am I crazy, or do I have a point? Hear me out for a minute, and then you can make the decision.

If you went into audiology because you wanted to help people, you are not alone. In fact, there are many professionals out there who want to fill that role. Chances are, you're not one of them because you have made it this far in the book. I have to assume that you, too, want more, that you want to grow your business, and you want to attain an even greater level of success. However, if owning your own business is not what you want, if it's just too much for you, and if you don't have the stamina to differentiate yourself and build the best hearing health care practice in your community, then I recommend you give me a call. I'll hire you as one of my associates, and you can spend your days clocking in and then heading home at night to do other things. This will allow you to have a job, do what is needed of you, go home at the end of the day, and leave the practice behind without having to worry about anything else. Someone else can take care of things while you are gone, and you can just continue to get your paycheck every week. Jeez! It doesn't get any easier than that!

But did you really get into the field to do that? I have a pretty good feeling you didn't. After all, you were crazy enough to become an entrepreneur. And I know you did it for the right reason—because you want to help as many people as possible and get paid well for being awesome. I know you want more than mediocrity because I have been where you are; I've experienced the stress, and now I can help others step up and grab the private practice bull by the horns!

The important thing you must realize is that the most successful providers and small business owners understand that they have countless roles that need to be managed. And this is in addition to being the main go-getter in their practice. If you desire a massively successful practice, you are going to have to wear many hats and take on many roles. You can't just manage patients all day, clock out at five, and head home. It doesn't work like that in the real world of an entrepreneur.

It doesn't work like that for me or anyone else in successful businesses that earn mid-seven or eight figures. And it never will. I'm also not suggesting that you must abandon yourself, your family, and your passion to work 16-hour days, seven days per week. What I'm saying is **work smarter, not harder**.

Are you thinking that means that you need to know how to run the reception desk, sweep the floors, and fix hearing issues all at the same time? Well, the answer is yes *and* no. You need to be hands-on in appointing the right people and putting the right systems in place in all areas of the practice. Once you get that all straightened out and have the right systems in place, you can go back to treating patients all day—or taking the day off to fly across the country to play in a charity golf event—and your office will continue to run as it should.

Or you can decide today to get into the business of constructing a system which automatically delivers patients to you by way of "magnetic attraction," where only the most qualified prospects come in and are elated to pay your fees without resistance because they understand the true value in being a patient at your practice. Luckily, you will also obtain rewards and success beyond what you can imagine once you get this right and join the top 1% in the profession.

Pound into your mind right now that **there is no single solution or easy button to get this done.** It takes true commitment to your success and the success of your practice.

Remove the notion of *easy* from your mind right now. You must fight its enticement because it simply doesn't exist for those who wish to create a successful business with true wealth, legacy, and epic retirement.

But I also want you to give up on the concept that this is going to be really hard. It doesn't have to be—but only if you have the right team and the right systems in place to make it happen.

If you want to achieve the level of success you really desire, you must have the right systems in place first. Are you ready to make the essential decisions to make that happen? Only you can take the steps to change your practice.

It is time to either take action to make it happen, be happy with averageness, or just leave the audiology field altogether. **The decision is completely up to you.**

ACTION ITEMS WHAT WILL YOU DO NEXT?

_____

_____

_____

_____

_____

_____

_____

_____

_____

_____

_____

_____

_____

_____

_____

_____

EPILOGUE
Looking Toward the Future

*"We are made wise not by the recollection of our past,
but by the responsibility for our future."*
—GEORGE BERNARD SHAW

NOW I KNOW THAT THERE IS NO WAY that you learned any of these things in professional school. I know because I didn't learn them either—and I went to business school! I have discovered these philosophies through painful trial and error and from researching some of the great business minds and businesses of our time. I have boiled the principles down and executed the most successful components in my own practices. Now my business runs exactly the way I want it to.

There isn't anything wrong with running things on your own terms, as long as you understand what business you are really in. When I finally converted my staff on the fact that we are not in the audiology business (thinking our only job was to work on ears) and got into the business of building relationships and forming a system that magnetically attracts patients to my practice, I saw the massive results that I had always dreamed of, minus the pains of more marketing, shady sales practices, or turning my staff into salesmen with high-pressure tactics taught by other practice management consultants. My life and my practice changed dramatically, and for the better. I finally began enjoying my practice life, I am able to spend more time with my kids, my staff is much more fulfilled, my patients give us higher approval ratings, and I do it all with just one day a week in the clinic.

I have no doubt that you can have this, too. I watched it happen, and I believe in sharing the secrets of my success with others. I have taken that to an assortment of levels, such as newsletters, seminars, books, and entire systems that can be put into place for your practice. I'd honestly love it for each and every one of you to achieve the level of success that I have, the level you truly want to have. There are certainly enough people with untreated hearing loss in our country to make this a reality (nearly 40,000,000 of them!).

I sincerely think that we have to produce the type of world we want by being active players. I can't sit around, watch my fellow colleagues in the audiology field struggle, and just continue down the road to my success without helping. The coach and problem solver in me simply won't permit that.

I have a great desire to share with you what it is that I know for a fact will make your practice every bit as successful as mine. I want you to start moving forward and thinking positively. Put the systems in place to make your practice really take off and reach the next level.

One of my favorites quotes is by Mithilesh Chudgar and say, "Be aware there is a gap between hopes and action. This gap is that of our fears, perceptions and inhibitions. Performing at the peak is about bridging this gap."

I have provided the tools to help you in bridging that gap and piloting your way. **Now you have to ask yourself if you will choose to use those tools.**

DISCOVER THE RENEGADE AUDIOLOGY MINDSET AND THE MOST INCREDIBLE FREE GIFTS

When You Claim Your Seat in Jared Brader's
Monthly Loud and Clear Program

L⊃UD AND CLEA[R]
MARKETING PROGRAM WITH JARED BRADE[R]

New Member
Roadmap Step 1

This marketing packet contains a complete marketing campaign that you can "swipe and deploy" in your own practice today.

The sample each month has been split-tested for headlines, photos, and offers. It has been proven to achieve at least a 5 to 1 return on investment in our practice.

Each month, in this letter, I bring you a sample marketing piece that has earned its place in the Intermountain Audiology marketing "hall of fame." One month it might be a direct mail piece, another month you might see a series of emails, landing pages, sales letters or even promotional contests we use in our office to stimulate referrals. Throughout the year, you might receive a tutorial on a single component of direct-response marketing (eg, headlines, offers, mailing list strategies, etc.)

Your job each month is to avoid saying "but this will never work in my practice." Instead you will ask yourself, "how can I make this work in my practice?" Serious students of mine are relentless tester of the marketing pieces I deliver each month. They are, incidentally, the audiologists with the highest net-incomes and highest satisfaction ratings in their current practices. There will always be a reason in your head why you don't want to try something new. The results come in **taking action**. I've made the path clearer for you, but there is no easy button.

ACCESS TO THE #1 AUDIOLOGY MARKETING PROGRAM
in North America where you will discover a new strategy each month that earns **5:1 or more return on investment** for our clinics and coaching clients.

PLUS GET THREE FREE REPORTS

guaranteed to impact your practice in meaningful and profitable ways you've never considered until now.

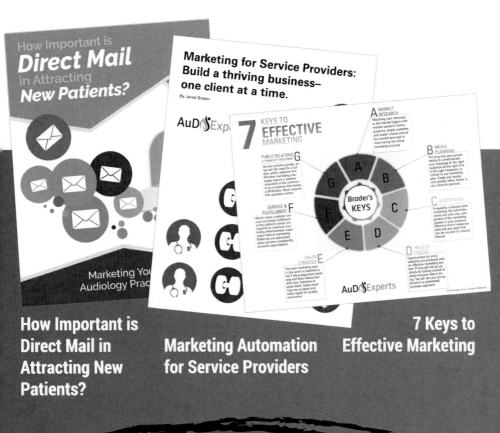

How Important is Direct Mail in Attracting New Patients?

Marketing Automation for Service Providers

7 Keys to Effective Marketing

SIGN UP TODAY AT
www.GreatAuDMarketing.com

Our vision is a world
where everyone can
experience the sound of life.

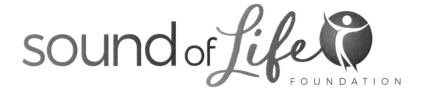

www.SoundOfLifeFoundation.org

Made in the USA
Lexington, KY
25 April 2018